CARSTEN REHBANN

Building Muscle at Home Made Easy

Simple strategies and hacks on how to build muscle and get shredded at home with ease and low time and money invest to maximize your success

This book was professionally typeset on Reedsy.
Find out more at reedsy.com

Contents

1

Introduction

Welcome to your companion on the journey to a lean and muscular body. Whether you're just starting out or, like me, have tried numerous paths in the past only to find yourself back at square one, this guide is for you. Over my 40 years, I've navigated different phases of life, each with its own set of challenges. But one goal has remained constant: to maintain my fitness. In my youth, I played American football, then I started training for and running marathons, eventually transitioning into fitness and strength training. I approached each endeavor with enthusiasm, trying out many different things. As a result, I also quit many things when they no longer fit into my life.

With three kids, one question became central to me: How can I stay fit and build a muscular body with minimal time investment, in a way that's flexible enough to fit my life, so I can stick with it no matter what?

This book doesn't offer pre-made workout or diet plans that are doomed to fail the moment they no longer fit into your life. Instead, it helps you easily create your own plan at home, one that's designed for your success.

We'll focus on the things that truly impact building a lean and muscular body. I'll also share a few hacks that you can integrate into your lifestyle, in a way that works for you.

So, let's get started…

2

The Issues With Classic Approaches

When it comes to fitness, muscle building, and the right nutrition, there's no shortage of information out there today. Science has also delved deeply into what positively affects muscle growth and how nutrition plays a role in that process. Keeping track of all this information can be overwhelming, and it raises a lot of questions. Which muscle groups should I train? Is full-body training better than split training? What machines do I need for the best results? Should I follow a low-carb, no-carb, keto, paleo, or some other type of diet?

Fortunately, there are countless guides and pre-made workout plans that have already taken these factors into account for you. You get precise instructions on which exercises to do during specific workouts and when to do them. Plus, there's a diet plan that tells you exactly what meals to eat and when.

However, you often realize that without a gym membership, you won't have access to the necessary equipment, so you have to invest time and money into that. Not everyone has a gym just around the corner, so travel time can easily add an extra 40 minutes or more to each workout (round trip). With pre-made diet plans, you might also find that some of the suggested foods don't appeal to your taste, or the portion sizes leave you feeling unsatisfied. Before you know it, you're skipping a workout because you'd rather go to a friend's party or attend your daughter's school play. When preparing meals, you might suddenly discover you're missing ingredients you've never heard of, and because you're still hungry, you end up snacking on the kids' leftovers or treating yourself to an extra protein bar.

Sure, you could boost your chances of success by hiring a personal fitness coach to help you navigate these obstacles. But that's not something everyone can afford.

Often, this ends with wasted time and money, without achieving the results you originally hoped for.

3

The Benefits of Home Workout

Training at home offers many advantages, with the most obvious being the savings in both time and money compared to a gym membership. You don't have to pay for an expensive membership, and you also save the time you'd spend traveling to and from the gym. Plus, you don't need costly or complicated equipment that requires instruction before you can start building muscle effectively. Anyone who has been to a gym has probably experienced the frustration of trying to work out during peak hours when certain machines are occupied right when you need them according to your training plan. That's something you won't have to worry about at home.

And when we talk about training at home, it doesn't just mean a room in your house or apartment. Since you need little to no equipment for a great workout, you can take your training to your hotel room while on vacation or business trips, or even to your backyard or a nearby park when the weather is nice. This flexibility has an added bonus - sunlight can positively impact your mood and energy levels.

For all these reasons, training at home can make it easier for you to stay consistent and reach your goal of building a muscular body.

4

What Equipment You Need

If you haven't trained much before and are just starting your muscle-building journey, you can achieve great results even without equipment. Later on, I'll recommend some bodyweight exercises that you can incorporate into your training plan to get started successfully right away.

However, to build muscle effectively, it's essential to gradually increase the intensity of your workouts to continuously challenge your muscles. This is the only way to stimulate growth. While you can achieve this by adding more sets, doing more repetitions, or training more frequently, you'll find that this approach has its limits. Incorporating additional equipment can help you make faster progress. This is especially important to consider if you've already been training and are in good shape.

Recommended Basic Equipment

Here's some equipment I recommend, as it can be purchased for a relatively low cost and will help you add resistance to all the key exercises needed for muscle building.

- **A Pair of Dumbbells**

  Dumbbells are great because they don't take up much space and are highly versatile. Plus, you know exactly how much weight you're lifting, allowing you to gradually increase it as you progress.

- **Resistance Bands**

  Resistance bands are very affordable and extremely space-efficient, making them easy to take with you when you travel. This means you can maintain your workout routine without any modifications, even when you're on vacation or on a business trip.

- **Suspension Trainer**

  Pull exercises are also crucial for building muscle, and a suspension trainer offers plenty of options for this. All you need is a door to set it up. Like resistance bands, a suspension trainer is compact and travel-friendly, so you can easily bring it along wherever you go.

Additional Equipment

The following equipment is especially helpful for basic exercises, though you can still make excellent progress without it.

- **Pull-Up Bar**

  If you have a sturdy door frame, there are models that can be easily hung there. However, a pull-up bar that is securely mounted to a wall or ceiling is more stable.

- **Barbell**

  A barbell is a great addition to your dumbbells, but it does require a bit more space.

- **Weight Bench**

  When choosing a weight bench, opt for a model with an adjustable backrest. This allows you to perform bench presses from various angles, adding variety to your workouts.

5

It Starts With Your "Why"

Before you dive in and start purchasing equipment that might end up collecting dust in the corner, it's important to take a step back. Beyond training and nutrition, there's another critical factor for your success: your "why." To succeed, you need to consistently stick to your plan, which means showing up for every single workout you've scheduled. There will be days when this feels incredibly challenging. Your inner voice might try to convince you that it's okay to skip just this one workout. But before you know it, that exception can become the rule. Having a strong "why" will help keep you motivated during these tough times and ensure you stay on track

The Reason Why YOU Bought This Book

What is your "why"? This is a question only you can answer, and it needs to be something so important to you that you're determined to stick with it no matter what. My "why" used to be about looking great, attracting women, and boosting my confidence. Nowadays, it's more about staying fit as I age and being a good role model for my kids. Your "why" can change over time, which is why it's crucial to think it through, write it down, and vividly imagine how it would feel to achieve it. The more clearly you can see, feel, and sense it, the better.

Find images of role models that inspire you. Look for YouTube videos that get you in a motivated mindset (personally, I love watching Arnold Schwarzenegger for this). For your brain, it doesn't matter if it's true yet or not—it will help you tap back into the initial motivation and feelings that got you started, especially during those tough times when sticking to your personal training plan feels like a struggle.

Type of Goals

Your "why" alone won't be enough to reach your goal. That brings us to an important topic: What exactly is your goal? It's crucial to be specific so that you can tailor your training and nutrition to achieve it. You need to know when you want to reach your goal and how you'll measure your success.

When you set clear, concrete goals, you'll be surprised at how naturally you start working toward them. Don't be surprised if you suddenly find time you didn't think you had - especially if your "why" is strong enough.

Don't limit yourself when setting goals. It's not just about hitting a certain weight on the scale by a specific date. There are plenty of other goals to consider.

For example, developing a new skill can be incredibly motivating. You might set a goal to do a certain number of pull-ups or handstand push-ups without assistance by a specific deadline.

Another type of goal could focus on behavior, like training for at least 20 minutes, four times a week, or consuming 1.5 to 2 grams of protein per kilogram of body weight each day.

When it comes to nutrition, setting positive goals can be more effective than restrictive ones. Instead of saying you won't eat sugar anymore, try setting a goal like eating at least one serving of fruit every day or stopping when you're full. Positive goals like these often lead to better success because restrictions can sometimes cause you to rebel against them and ultimately fail to stick to them.

The Right Approach For You

Not all of us start out with the ambition to become Mr. Universe, and everyone has different circumstances. The most important thing is to find an approach that fits your life and allows you to stay consistent. You'll be more successful if you stick with something slow but steady rather than pushing through an intense program for a short time only to burn out and quit.

Develop a plan that is realistic for you and adjust it if necessary, rather than starting without a plan or following one that doesn't suit your lifestyle. The advantage of a plan that fits your life and goals is that you build routines you can easily stick to, without having to think too much about what comes next.

How to Make Your Success Measurable

When it comes to building muscle, it's important to track your progress and measure the right things. The number on the scale isn't it, because as your muscle mass increases, so will your weight—muscle weighs more than fat. The scale doesn't tell you whether weight gain is from muscle or fat. It's more useful to measure your biceps, chest, and waist with a tape measure. Also, comparison photos of your body can be very motivating when you see how positively you've changed over time.

To keep track of whether your training and diet are on plan, it's essential to maintain a workout and nutrition journal. I used to think I didn't need one. I knew how many reps I did with what weight last time, and I remembered what I ate during the day. But I quickly realized I was wrong when I had to think about how much weight to put on the bar before starting a set or how many extra calories were in that candy bar I hadn't even considered a snack. Especially for tracking your diet, there are good, free apps that can help. It may seem tedious at first, but as you get into a routine, it becomes easier and will help you stay on track with your nutrition.

6

What Really Counts When You Want to Build Muscle

Build muscle and get shredded at once?

If you're a complete beginner, it's possible to build muscle and look more defined at the same time. This is because regular training helps your body more easily switch into fat-burning mode after a workout. Plus, the muscles you're building—especially in the beginning—burn more calories, even when your body is at rest.

However, as you progress, this isn't the case anymore. To build more muscle, your body needs a calorie surplus. This allows for muscle growth but also means some of those excess calories will be stored as fat. That's why bodybuilding typically involves two phases. First, there's the muscle-building phase, where the goal is to maximize muscle growth. As a competition approaches, athletes switch to a phase focused on looking more defined and reducing body fat. Which phase you're in affects how you design your training and nutrition plan.

So, if you already have some experience with strength training, you should decide whether you want to focus more on building muscle or getting a defined body. For me, I had a few extra pounds that bothered me, so my first step was to reduce my body fat percentage, even if that meant making slower progress on muscle gains initially.

Early or Late Training?

Whether you train in the morning or evening won't make a direct difference in your muscle growth. Both have their pros and cons, and you should consider these when creating your plan. The key is to choose what helps you stay consistent.

For example, morning workouts often leave you feeling more energized and happier throughout the day. Since you've already completed your workout, there's less chance something will come up in the afternoon or evening that could force you to skip it. Morning exercise can also positively impact your sleep quality, which is important for fat burning and recovery. However, night owls who find it hard to wake up early might struggle with morning workouts. Another downside is that your body isn't at peak performance in the morning.

On the other hand, you can benefit from your body's higher performance levels in the evening. You might also have less time pressure at night since there are no more appointments. Plus, a tough workout can help you release the frustrations of a bad workday. However, there's a greater risk of feeling too tired in the evening, which might tempt you to skip your workout. Social distractions, like going out with colleagues, can also interfere. Additionally, intense evening workouts might make it harder for you to fall asleep.

Keeping these pros and cons in mind, you should decide when it's easiest for you to schedule your workouts. Block that time in your calendar, so it's easier to stick to. And by the way, there's nothing wrong with squeezing in a workout during your lunch break if, for example, you have the option to work from home.

A Focused Mind

Your body does the work, but what many people overlook is the importance of mental focus. You often see people at the gym chatting, on the phone, or watching TV. The result is that their breaks between sets get longer, the intensity of their exercises drops, or they lose their form. This can keep you from getting the results you could achieve.

When you train, it's important to focus on your workout and avoid distractions. Listening to music that motivates you and blocks out external distractions can help.

Another way to enhance your training is by focusing on your mind-muscle connection. This means concentrating on the muscles you're targeting during an exercise and trying to feel them working. For example, when doing bench presses, focus on your chest muscles and feel them contract as you lower the weight. You can also slow down the movement when lowering the weight. This increases the time the muscle is under tension and allows you to feel it more. It also helps you practice proper form.

This focus on what you're doing in your training is an easy way to get more out of your workout compared to just going through the motions. Additionally, it improves your mindfulness in general, helping you stay present in the moment. The positive effects can extend beyond just your training success. You can also apply this focus to eating. Many people eat on the go or while multitasking to save time, but focusing on your food—chewing thoroughly and noticing the flavors—can help you recognize when you're full. This is especially helpful when you're aiming for a more defined body, as it reduces the likelihood of overeating or mindlessly snacking.

How to Ensure Progress?

To make progress, it's essential that you continuously challenge yourself in your workouts. If you keep doing the same routine with the same number of repetitions without increasing the weight or resistance, your workouts may become easier, but your muscles won't grow. For muscle growth to occur, you need to create a stimulus, and as you build more muscle, you'll need to do more to trigger further growth. This concept is known as progressive overload.

Most people think of increasing weight when they hear progressive overload, but you can achieve it in other ways too. You can increase the number of reps or sets, train more frequently each week, or focus on performing reps with better technique. The goal is to improve with every workout.

n the beginning, it's easier to make progress with each session. However, the longer you train, the harder it becomes. Instead of getting frustrated when you hit a plateau with weight or resistance, consider other methods of progressive overload to continue making progress.

For beginners, it's advisable to start with lighter weights or resistance and focus more on proper form. Performing exercises more slowly can also help improve technique.

Success Killers

There are factors that can negatively affect your training success. For example, you should plan recovery days, which are essential for actual muscle growth and preventing overtraining. Overtraining can lead to injuries and prevent you from regaining the energy and strength needed for further progress.

Poor or insufficient sleep can also have a negative impact. Aim for 7 to 8 hours of sleep each night. Avoid caffeine in the late evening and too much alcohol, as both can disrupt your sleep and reduce your energy levels.

Once you've established your training plan, resist the urge to constantly change it or swap exercises. Stick to your plan for at least 6 to 8 weeks, and longer if you're still making progress. This consistency allows you to track your progress in your training journal and recognize when it's time to introduce new stimuli through a new training plan.

Focus on the "Big Six"

There are exercises that target multiple muscle groups at once, allowing you to train your entire body with just six exercises. These foundational exercises are especially effective for beginners who can achieve quick results by focusing on them during each session. Additionally, these exercises offer an efficient workout that can be completed in a short amount of time. You can complete one round of all six exercises with 12 reps each, followed by a 2-minute break and a second round, in just 20 minutes, providing an effective workout.

Advanced lifters should not only focus on the Big Six but also incorporate isolation exercises (e.g., bicep curls, standing calf raises, sit-ups) into their training plan to target specific muscles. However, it's beneficial to include one or two of the Big Six in every session as foundational exercises.

The Big Six include the following exercises:

- **Squats**
  Squats can be performed with or without weights or resistance bands, allowing you to easily increase intensity to target the lower body and core.
- **Bench Press**
  The bench press is a classic weightlifting exercise that can be done in various forms. An alternative without weights is push-ups, which can also be performed in different variations to effectively train the chest and triceps with different focuses.
- **Barbell/Dumbbell Rows**
  Barbell rows primarily target the upper back, with weights or resistance bands. Suspension trainers or even filled water bottles can serve as alternatives.
- **Deadlifts**
  Deadlifts mainly work the lower body and lower back. The intensity can be increased with weights or resistance bands. Bodyweight exercises like good mornings are an alternative that can be done without weights.
- **Pull-ups**
  Pull-ups can be challenging for beginners, with some struggling to perform even one. In such cases, resistance bands can be used to reduce your body weight. Alternatively, you can do rows using the edge of a sturdy table. Suspension trainers also offer excellent alternatives with varying difficulty levels.

- **Military Press**
  This exercise targets the shoulders, with intensity increased through weights or resistance bands. Lateral raises with filled water bottles can be an alternative.

Full Body Workout or Split Training

There are different approaches to creating a workout plan. The simplest is a full-body workout in each session, where you target all muscle groups in one workout. This approach works well with fewer sessions per week and ensures that all muscle groups are trained. Its simplicity makes it ideal for beginners.

Then, there are various forms of split training. In split training, you focus on specific muscle groups in each session, ensuring that all muscle groups are trained over the course of a week. This method is great if you can fit in more sessions per week but have limited time per session. Common splits include:

- Upper body/Lower body
- Push exercises/Pull exercises/Legs
- Chest/Back/Shoulders/Legs/Arms/2 Rest Days

For advanced lifters, split training allows for higher intensity by focusing on fewer muscle groups per session. Additionally, the muscle groups have more time to recover before the next intense session.

Regardless of the approach you choose, all of them can effectively build muscle. It's more important to choose a plan that fits your weekly schedule in terms of the number of sessions and the time available per session. The key is to stick to a plan that makes it easier for you to stay consistent.

Impact of Your Diet

Nutrition is also a crucial factor in building muscle. As mentioned earlier, it's important to know your current focus: Do you want to lose weight and achieve a lean physique, or are you primarily aiming for muscle growth? Your body burns calories to keep running, which you consume through your diet. If you consume fewer calories than your body needs, you'll lose weight. If you consistently consume more, you'll gain weight.

Calories come from three sources, known as macronutrients. Carbohydrates are the easiest for the body to burn and are preferred during workouts because they provide quick energy. It can be helpful to have a carbohydrate snack 30 minutes before a workout if you haven't eaten for several hours. The second source of energy is protein, which is essential for muscle building. When carbohydrate stores are depleted, the body turns to protein for quick energy. The third source is fat, which is the hardest for the body to burn. The body relies on fat during rest periods or light activity. Adequate and good sleep also promotes fat burning.

If you're in a calorie deficit and training regularly, your body will build less muscle but will primarily use fat reserves for energy instead of protein, which would lead to muscle breakdown if you weren't training. On the other hand, if you consume more calories and train, your body will use the extra calories to build muscle, as long as you're getting enough protein. However, you will also gain some fat, although the muscle gain will outweigh the fat gain.

Understanding these concepts is important, which is why tracking your diet is essential. This is the only way to ensure you're getting the right amount of calories and sufficient protein to build muscle.

Which Supplements Can Help Improve My Progress?

In general, you can get all the nutrients you need from food. However, three supplements can be helpful for muscle building:

Protein Shakes

Meeting your protein needs for muscle building can sometimes be difficult through diet alone. Protein shakes offer an easy solution. Protein powder is versatile and can be used to enhance meals. For example, mix some quark with a little milk and two scoops of protein powder, add fresh fruit like blueberries, and you have a quick, easy snack.

Magnesium

Magnesium supports muscle recovery, especially if you're prone to muscle cramps. Look for a supplement where magnesium citrate is the main ingredient, as the body absorbs this form well. Cheaper products often contain magnesium oxide, which is harder for the body to process.

Creatine

Creatine helps your muscles produce more energy for short bursts, allowing you to complete that one extra rep that increases the training stimulus. It's also beneficial for brain function. While creatine isn't a game-changer, it's well-researched for its positive effects and is a good addition to your regimen.

7

Make It Work For You

After going through the previous chapters, you now have a basic understanding of what is essential for building muscle successfully and the key factors you can leverage. The next step is to create your personalized plan. Many people think they don't need a plan because they already know the basics: train more and watch your diet a little. They believe they can do it without a plan. I've had phases where I approached it this way, but I quickly realized that I wasn't making progress and, at best, wasn't gaining weight.

The point is, you are making a change in your life, and changes are never automatic—they require mental effort, especially at the beginning. The longer you stick with it, the more likely it will become a routine that keeps you on track almost effortlessly. But first, you need to get to that point. A plan helps by reducing the number of decisions you have to make and eliminates the need to think about what to do next. All you have to do is follow your plan, which significantly reduces the chances of making poor decisions or giving up. Additionally, a plan allows you to track your progress, and if you're not making progress, you can identify areas that may need adjustments to get you back on track.

How to Build Your Own Training Routine and Plan

First, look at which days you can realistically schedule your workouts and fit them into your daily routine. Consider how much time you can dedicate to each session. Choose the number of days and times that are realistic for you to stick to. This helps avoid skipping sessions, especially at the beginning. Over time, your training will likely become a higher priority, making it easier to increase workout times or add sessions. However, when starting, focus on what you can realistically manage.

Your Training Schedule for the Week

The minimum is three 30-minute sessions or two 45-minute sessions per week (plus the time it takes to freshen up after training) to see results. If you're more advanced, you should plan for more time or more sessions to incorporate progressions, such as more repetitions or sets.

Based on the number of sessions and the time available per session, decide whether you want to do full-body workouts or follow a split-training plan. If you have fewer sessions but more time, a full-body workout is recommended. If you have more sessions with fewer rest days and shorter workout times, a split-training plan might be more suitable.

An example of a simple weekly plan with a full-body workout could look like this:

- **Mon**: Full-body - 45 Min.
- **Tue**: Rest

- **Wed**: Full-body - 45 Min.
- **Thu**: Rest
- **Fri**: Full-body - 45 Min.
- **Sat**: Rest
- **Sun**: Rest

Alternatively, with different training days and times, your weekly plan with a split-training plan and one full-body day might look like this:

- **Mon**: Chest- 30 Min.
- **Tue**: Rest
- **Wed**: Back - 30 Min.
- **Thu**: Legs - 30 Min.
- **Fri**: Rest
- **Sat**: Full-body - 60 Min.
- **Sun**: Rest

As you can see, you can easily create a flexible training plan that fits into your week.

Pick Your Exercises

The foundation of your training sessions should always be exercises from the "Big Six." These exercises alone are enough for an effective full-body workout. For example, if you have at least one rest day between workout days, a simple full-body workout plan for a beginner might be:

Round 1:

- Set 1: Squats, 12 reps
- Set 2: Push-ups, 12 reps

- Set 3: Pull-ups, 12 reps
- Set 4: Dumbbell Rows, 12 reps
- Set 5: Deadlifts, 12 reps
- Set 6: Military Press, 12 reps

Rest for 2 minutes

Round 2:

- Repeat all exercises from Round 1

Rest for 2 minutes

Round 3 (optional, if time allows):

- Repeat all exercises from Round 1

For split training, always base your sessions on the "Big Six" exercises that target the muscle groups you're focusing on. Add other exercises to complement these primary exercises for the muscle groups you're targeting. You'll find plenty of exercises online for each muscle group, so choose ones you can perform with your available equipment.

For example, a selection of exercises for leg day might include:

- Squats as a base exercise
- Lunges
- Back Lunges
- Step-ups
- Standing Calf Raises

These exercises have the advantage of being performed with or without weights or resistance bands, which is helpful if you find yourself without equipment while traveling. You can still complete your workout.

Find good instructional videos for all exercises—these are easy to find online. A good video explains the individual phases of a movement and highlights important points to ensure proper technique. Do this for each exercise, even if you think you already know how to do them. Proper technique is crucial for making progress and avoiding injury. During the first few workouts, focus on executing the exercises correctly. Start with lighter weights or resistance. The initial sessions will also help determine the weight/resistance, repetitions, and sets you should begin with. Aim to challenge your muscles, with your repetitions starting between 8 and 14 per set.

Making Progress - Options to Increase Intensity

If you perform the same sets and repetitions, use the same weights/resistance, and take the same rest periods during each workout, your progress will eventually plateau. To continue making progress, you need to increase the intensity over time.

The easiest way is to gradually increase the weight or resistance. If you're doing bodyweight exercises, you can aim to complete more repetitions within a set time (e.g., 45 seconds). As a beginner, you'll progress quickly, but this becomes more challenging as you advance.

There are also other methods. You can aim to add one more repetition per set. For example, if you can do 10 reps with a certain weight, try to do 11 next time, until you reach 14 reps. Then, increase the weight and start again at the number of reps you can handle with the new weight.

Another way to increase intensity is by shortening the rest periods between sets, which gives your muscles less time to recover. You can also add an additional set to your workouts. Instead of three sets, perform four and go to muscle failure on the last set, doing as many reps as you can until you can't complete another.

If you can, consider adding another workout session on an extra day to increase your training volume.

If you hit a plateau, where progress seems to stall, you can experiment with these methods. However, if you're overloading your muscles too much and not making progress, you might need to schedule more rest or reduce the weights for a few sessions to focus on correct technique.

How to Improve Your Diet Routines

First, clarify your primary goal. Do you want to focus on building a defined body and losing fat, or is your main focus muscle building?

The answer is important to determine how many calories you should consume daily to reach your goal. Use an online calorie calculator for bodybuilding to determine your daily caloric needs based on a few inputs.

Since it's hard to estimate the calorie and macronutrient content of your meals, you should also start a food diary to track your nutrition. There are great apps that make tracking easy.

Radically changing your diet overnight often leads to frustration and reverting to old habits. Instead, make gradual changes and develop routines that become second nature.

To build muscle, you need protein. A high-protein diet also helps prevent cravings, so aim for about 1.5 to 2 grams of protein per kilogram of body weight. For example, at 80 kg, you should aim to consume 120 to 160 grams of protein per day. You can achieve this through protein-rich foods, but if you follow a vegetarian diet or are focused on building a defined body, it might be challenging. Protein powder is a great option to meet your protein needs, whether through shakes, adding it to yogurt, or preparing tasty desserts with protein powder.

A good starting point is to assess your current diet. Then, think about changes you can make that fit easily into your daily routine.

Here are some examples of changes you can make:

- Instead of sugary desserts, opt for yogurt or Skyr with protein powder.
- Start every morning and every meal with a large glass of water to feel fuller faster and eat less.
- Eat carbohydrate-rich foods in the morning or about 30 minutes before a workout when your body burns them more efficiently. The time spent sleeping and after your workout is better utilized for fat burning.
- Intermittent fasting is a dietary approach that's good for fat burning and easy to integrate into your daily routine - simply skip breakfast or dinner.
- If you need to consume more calories for muscle growth, nuts are a great source of healthy extra calories.
- If you usually snack on chocolate bars, switch to protein bars instead.
- Make a shopping list before you go to the store and stick to it to avoid impulse buying unhealthy snacks or foods.

- Incorporate more high-protein vegetables like beans and lentils into your meals. You can find plenty of options online and choose the ones you like. The more colorful, the better.
- Prepare a container of chopped fruits or vegetables every morning and try to snack on them throughout the day.
- On Sundays, prep your meals for the workweek if you don't have time to cook during the week. This way, you'll have ready meals and won't resort to fast food.
- Many calories come from sugary drinks. Drink water or unsweetened teas instead. Opt for sugar-free drinks when you crave something sweet. Low-sugar options are available in many places.
- Before every meal, ask yourself, "How much protein is in this?" You should eat foods that contain protein with every meal.

These are just a few possibilities. You can find numerous tips on the internet. Try to integrate things into your life that work for you and make it your goal to gradually develop healthy routines. You can also make it fun by choosing one change and then writing a smiley face in a calendar for each day you stick to it. The aim is "Don't break your chain" and to have as many smiley faces in a row as possible. As a reward, you could treat yourself to a visit to the spa after a successful month, for example.

Don't think of these dietary changes as sacrifices or drastic adjustments; instead, find what works for you and start making small changes. Over time, you'll develop healthy habits that are easy to follow. There will still be days when you treat yourself to something, but don't worry about it; just keep going with your plan.

Ultimately, it is important for your muscle building goal that you reach your daily calorie target and the required amount of protein. To do this, it is important to track your diet and gradually make the changes in your life that will help you achieve your nutritional goals.

8

Conclusion

After reading this book, you now know which aspects are important for successfully building a defined and muscular body. You don't need ready-made plans or a strict recipe and diet plan that don't fit into your life and are therefore doomed to failure. You should now be able to create a plan on your own that you can integrate into your life and how you can gradually expand and adapt it. This is how you create your success with gradual changes. The most important thing is that you keep at it, and a plan that makes it easy for you to do this will help you to do so. You can find a lot more helpful information on the subject and spend hours familiarizing yourself with it. But at this point, you already know everything you need to get started.

So take action now and start your transformation to a defined and muscular body.

Your Carsten

www.ingramcontent.com/pod-product-compliance
Lightning Source LLC
Chambersburg PA
CBHW061546250726
48657CB00006B/2317